Treatments for Tremors

Natural Therapies to Calm Tremors

What are possible causes of tremors? What natural remedies can help to calm them? A variety of natural therapies are presented that have proven useful for sedating tremors. These include supplements, essential oils, herbs, foods, aroma therapy, stress reduction, trauma release, sound therapy, vibration therapy, energy healing, transformation of beliefs and activating the limitless power of the mind. The key to success is taking control of the tremor rather than allowing the tremor to control you.

Treatments for Tremors

Contents

© Parkinsons Recovery

Treatments for Tremors

Treatments for Tremors

Treatments for Tremors

Treatments for Tremors

Introduction

After a decade of conducting research on the factors that offer the opportunity to reverse symptoms of Parkinson's disease I have drawn one key conclusion: The key to recovery is to maintain control over the physical, emotional and mental challenges that are confronted day in and day out. As soon as someone else or something else gets in the driver's seat, symptoms will inevitably escalate. Prospects for reversing symptoms are excellent as long as you are in control of any and all decisions that are made about your health.

The therapies I have included in this book are designed to put you in the driver's seat. You maintain control over your own recovery. Some therapies require instruction from a practitioner, but once the technique has been learned and practiced it can be accessed any time when it is needed. Ability to control your tremor resides entirely within your control.

Take Charge of Your Tremor

Professional Dancer Pamela Quinn[1] uses some counter intuitive approaches to control her own tremor. She does

---

[1] http://www.pamelaquinn.net

Treatments for Tremors

not let the tremor control her. Rather, she always maintains control:

> *I take charge of the tremor. I shake the tremor. I don't let the tremor shake me. I do it. That way I am manipulating it. I am taking control of it. There is this sort of psychological benefit as well as a physical one.*
>
> *Then, when I release my arm the muscles are relaxed for a bit. The tremor won't go away totally. It will come back. Then I do that again.*
>
> *If I am in a social situation where I do not want to look like a crazy person shaking my body around - I will put my hand under my leg. When my tremor starts up I shift position. I will put my hand on my hip or behind my back. If my tremor starts up I will shift it again. I will even sit on my hands.*
>
> *As soon as my body enters a physical behavior that I don't want I interrupt it and I shift to another mode. That is a way of saying "No. I am not going there."*

Treatments for Tremors

Three Options for Treating Tremors

Tremors can be suppressed by a wide variety of therapies. Prescription medications can get the problem under control for several years or longer. Natural herbs have proven beneficial to many persons. Exercise always creates endorphins which are the magical gateway to feeling delicious inside.

When using treatments such as medicines and supplements to suppress tremors and other symptoms, higher dosages taken more frequently are usually necessary to achieve the same effect over time. Some people are able to continue low dosages for many years. For others, the time before dosage has to be increased equates to months, not years. Everyone responds differently to medicines and supplements.

At some point, effectiveness plateaus. Increases in dosage have no effect on calming the tremors. Some people choose Deep Brain Stimulation (DBS) surgery as an option. This is recommended for some people who get diminishing returns from taker higher and higher doses of medications.

© Parkinsons Recovery

Treatments for Tremors

DBS suppresses tremors and other symptoms with less medication for some people.

Unintended consequences are experienced when the body becomes overwhelmed with having to process the waste from the substances that are ingested. These substances include supplements, herbs, essential oils and, of course, prescription medications. These unintended consequences are otherwise known as side effects. The addition of any additional substance – even food – can shift the body's capacity to function into overdrive as it nears the tipping point of a functional breakdown.

Why? The body has a limited capacity to "digest" what is swallowed and sent to the stomach. It is fully capable of eliminating waste and toxins. Eliminating toxins is one of its primary functions and responsibilities. When the quantity and toxicity are too much to process, the body's capacity to eliminate the toxins gets log jammed. Toxins build up in the tissues and organs. The result is a feeling of sluggishness and overwhelm. Tremors flare. New, unwanted symptoms inevitably develop. Tremors become only one of many other irritating problems to solve.

Treatments for Tremors

Everyone makes three choices about how to calm their tremors day in and day out, moment to moment.

1. Suppress the tremors.
2. Treat the cause(s).
3. Pursue both strategies.

I have concluded it makes the most sense to pursue both strategies: i.e. pursue the 3rd option: Suppress symptoms and, at the same time, address the cause. Both approaches are discussed in this book. Instead of focusing all of your energy and resources on racing to find one therapy or another that offers the promise of suppressing tremors, I recommend that you allocate some of your scarce and precious energy initially to exploring the causes. A combination of problems is usually implicated when tremors are symptomatic.

It is also important to find therapies that suppress tremors at least temporarily for one important reason. The tremors themselves create unrelenting stress in the body. When stress escalates, tremors become more pronounced. The cycle is endless as tremors cause more and more stress in the body. Heightened stress aggravates tremors which eventually burst into earthquake mode.

Think of your body as your "best friend". Your "best friend" – i.e., your body – is tremoring. Your body is making a serious attempt to communicate with you. Pay attention here! Imbalances need to be corrected. Your "best friend" needs a helping hand and a little loving care. What is out of balance? How can it be addressed?

Evidence of tremors is priceless information your "best friend" is conveying to you. They cannot fix this problem without help. You would rush to help a "best friend" who is in trouble and cannot solve it themselves, wouldn't you? Why not serve the needs of the most important "best friend" throughout your lifetime – your own body?

Adopt a Healthy Perspective

Most people who experience tremors see them as a horrible nuisance. On one level of course that is precisely what they are – a nuisance! Recovery from Parkinson's disease, or an essential tremor or whatever the diagnosis for the tremor happens to be – means that you have successfully eradicated the tremor or, at a minimum, numbed your neurological system so that the tremor does not exist.

There is an alternative mindset that some people have pursued to great advantage. Professional photographer Alan Babbitt has discovered that his tremor offers a creative advantage. Instead of trying to still his hand when he takes pictures, Alan allows his camera to jiggle in whatever position his hands move. He has produced a remarkable series of pictures that he aptly describes as "tremor enhanced" work. The images are incredible in every respect. I was so struck by Alan's photography that I purchased the rights to use one of Alan's "tremor enhanced" images as the featured cover of my book, *Road to Recovery from Parkinsons Disease*.[2]

A second person with Parkinson's who has used his tremor to great advantage is Whit Deschner. Whit is the founder of the Salt Lick contest in Baker City, Oregon which raises money for Parkinson's research every year. Whit has been a featured guest on my radio show.[3] How does author and

[2] http://www.parkinsonsdisease.me

[3] http://www.blogtalkradio.com/parkinsons-

Treatments for Tremors

humorist Whit Deschner uses his tremor to great advantage?

I have no doubt there are many answers to this question, given Whit's off the chart creativity, humor and innovativeness. Like Alan Babbitt, Whit has found his tremor to be of immense advantage in his own photography. Whit's approach differs from Alan's however.

Whit has always loved to take pictures, especially pictures of children as they jump. After experiencing the symptoms of Parkinson's, Whit found that when he began taking a picture of a child jumping his finger continued to snap the shot because of his tremor. Instead of capturing one image he would invariably wind up with a series of single shots taken with his still camera.

What do you do with a series of single shots of the same scene? Choose the "best"? Or, why not arrange them all in a sequence of slide show like images. When you string together the images together in a sequence, it looks much

recovery/2011/08/17/salt-lick

12

Treatments for Tremors

like a movie of the scene such as a child jumping. Talk about being creative!

There is a YouTube video tells the history of horses on Whit's ranch. It is well worth taking 9 minutes of time to watch this inspirational (and very entertaining) video[4]. When you watch, pay particular attention to the segments where you see evidence of Whit using all of the images from a still camera. Instead of seeing a still picture, you see a horse gracefully moving through a pasture or smiling back at you with a sweet grin on their face. There is no mention of how Whit Deschner has used to advantage his tremor in this video, but I wanted you to know.

To summarize, some people think of tremors of a liability. Other people - like Whit and Alan - think of tremors as an asset which has led to remarkable discoveries and innovations. It is a choice for everyone.

---

[4] http://www.youtube.com/watch?v=MB2HlLhRZjU

Treatments for Tremors

What Causes Tremors?

Most people believe that when they get a confirmation of a cause for their tremors – such as the presence of mercury – allocating all of their scarce resources and energy on detoxing mercury from their body will be all that is necessary. For most people unfortunately, the journey to heal the cause of tremors requires a much more comprehensive strategy. Yes, mercury may most clearly be a causative factor, but it is likely only one among other factors that are causing the problem of tremors.

A variety of conditions in the body can and do cause tremors. They also usually work in combination to provoke synergetic effects. The impact of two conditions taken together can be far greater than the impact of any one that is considered independent of the other. I recommend you consider the possibility that more than one cause applies to your own situation.

My short list of potential causes for tremors include the following: stress, alcoholism, toxins and critters (such as bacterial infections and parasites). Any one of these can play a role – either a major role or a supporting one – and

14

work in combination with others to cause tremors to be even more intense.

Stress

My research reveals one consistent pattern. Tremors are anything but constant. The intensity varies considerably over the course of a single day. The extent to which the tremors become "out of control" is no accident.

Stress clearly plays a leading role in the drama. When people are stressed, tremors do flare up. An overwhelm soaks into the tissues of the body. The more you try to wrestle with a stressful situation, the worse the tremors become. When you spar with stress, you are never victorious.

Stressful situations equate to intense tremors. Less stressful situations are associated with mild or nonexistent tremors. More succinctly, the more intense the stress, the worse is the tremor. The situation escalates into a vicious downward cycle. If your tremors are flaring up, it is a smart practice to accept the reality of your present situation: You are stressed out!

Treatments for Tremors

- Most people do not realize how stressful their lives really are.
- Most people deal with extremely stressful situations stress every day.
- Most people numb themselves to the damage that is being done to their physical body from stress.

Worst of all, most people may not even be aware their stress level is about to burst the pressure valve that is already set on the highest level that is physically tolerable. Without a release valve of some type – like a practice of mindfulness or Tai Chi or Qigong – tremors will escalate.

Alcoholism

In my own family system, many ancestors and family members have been cursed with addiction to alcoholism and drugs. Family members died at a very early age because they could not stop drinking or drugging. I have had the unfortunate opportunity to observe the horrible consequences of addiction time and time again:

- Hands shake uncontrollably.
- Heads shake from side to side.
- Legs become restless.

© Parkinsons Recovery

Treatments for Tremors

- Bodies shiver from top to bottom.

Has excessive drinking of alcohol or drugging been an issue for you? If so, there is only one treatment that offers you the opportunity to silence your tremors. The addictive behavior must be confronted head on. You can experiment with the many suggestions offered in my book, but none of them will succeed until and unless you stop drinking and/or drugging.

Alcoholic drinks contain excessive toxins, as do street drugs. If you persist in drinking alcoholic beverages on a regular basis, your body will eventually be unable to process the back log of toxins. Alcohol also strips bare the myelin sheaths that cover neurons. Tremors that result will ultimately lead to horrendous consequences: loss of jobs, loss of mobility and loss of independence.

Toxins

To what extent have you been exposed to dangerous toxins of one type or another?

- *How about exposure to Agent Orange?*
- *How about exposure to radiation?*

© Parkinsons Recovery

Treatments for Tremors

- *How about exposure to pesticides?*
- *How about exposure to heavy metals?*
- *How about exposure to electromagnetic pollution?*

If your answer is "yes" to any of the above questions, make detoxing a lifelong priority in your life. Tremors will remain a problem until you do.

Perhaps your answer is "no" to these questions. If so, I suspect you are in denial. Perhaps our ancestors could answer "no" to these questions and be correct. Today we all live in a very, very toxic world. We are all subjected to toxins every day. Do you use a cell phone? My case rests.

Critters

Unwelcome critters in the form of bacteria and viruses – there are so many possibilities here – can live inside your body and cause neurological havoc.

1. *Is Lyme disease a possible factor for you? Symptoms of Lyme are the same as those of Parkinson's.*

2. *Do you have an overgrowth of candida? This can cause Parkinson's symptoms too.*

3. *Is it possible that you have a reaction to a tetanus inoculation? Sharry Edwards[5] has found that tetanus is a causative factor for a surprising number of people who have had her BioAcoustic profiling done.*

Summary

When your only strategy is to suppress symptoms, the therapies you have chosen will have to be continued year in and year out. The cause is unknown and untreated.

Finding and treating the cause of tremors promises the potential for long lasting relief. When your body stops tremoring, you will know that the cause of the imbalances have been found and healed. There will no longer be a need to suppress the tremors. Ask:

> *What is the underlying cause of my tremors?*
> *What is the tremor telling me in the moment?*

---

[5] http://www.soundhealthoptions.com

© Parkinsons Recovery

Treatments for Tremors

Herbs, medicines and other natural treatments can and do suppress tremors temporarily. But, if you want tremors to be suppressed permanently – you will need to put your recovery plan on pause. Step back from yourself. Set the intention to find the cause of your tremor:

- *Perhaps you are under extreme stress. Your body is telling you to slow down, change jobs or chill out.*
- *Perhaps you are using a soap or detergent that is toxic.*
- *Perhaps you are being exposed day in and day out to electromagnetic pollution from use of a hybrid car or "smart" electrical meter.*
- *Perhaps you have a low level infection.*
- *Perhaps …*

Yes. The list of possible causes is long and overwhelming in itself. Once you determine the factor (or factors) that cause your tremors, a viable resolution can be found. Best of all, once the cause has been identified and treated you no longer need to suppress the shaking (or tremor) with a drug, herb, supplement, food or other therapy.

© Parkinsons Recovery

Treatments for Tremors

The method for identifying causes of illness I have personally used and found useful is the bioenergetic assessment. This holistic method for assessing imbalances in the body is discussed in my book: *What is Wrong with Me?* [6]

---

[6]

http://www.amazon.com/gp/product/1508516812/ref=as_li_tl?ie=UTF8&camp=1789&creative=9325&creativeASIN=1508516812&linkCode=as2&tag=zerpoihea-20&linkId=JTT5GOGU4AEDNF4M

Treatments for Tremors

How do I Decide?

I am guessing you wanted to read my book, *Treatments for Tremors*, with the anticipation that there would be a few therapies at best that might potentially help calm your tremor. I have my first surprise for you! There are not just a few options. There are many! Best of all, each is useful to one extent or another.

The challenge is to figure out which therapies are worth spending your time, money and energy on. I have a framework for you to consider that helps prioritize and guide the therapies you wind up exploring further and perhaps even deciding to try.

Some people prefer to focus on only one treatment or therapy at a time. They want to know whether the therapy helps or not. My observation from researching Parkinson's disease for more than a decade is that a combination of therapies offers the best opportunity to see good results. Consider playing the odds of getting good results by pursing more than one therapy at the same time. This will maximize the possibility you have the tool set that you need to calm tremors whenever sedation is needed.

© Parkinsons Recovery

Treatments for Tremors

Everyone has a unique body. You cannot be certain at the outset of any recovery protocol that will offer the most beneficial outcome. My "hedge your bets" strategy is analogous to horse race betting. You will be more likely to win if you place bets on more than one horse to win (or show or place).

My "hedge your bets" strategy is also what most parents do when helping a child settle down at bedtime. Pacifiers work, but not every night. Reading a book to a child helps, but not every night. Rocking the child to sleep helps, but not every night.

I predict you will get the best results with sedating your tremor if you have one treatment or therapy in your "tremor sedation tool kit" that capitalizes on addressing more than one of the following intentions:

- Reduce Stress
- Move Your Body Gently
- Release Trauma
- Take Supplements and/or Herbs
- Eat Wisely
- Relax with Aroma Therapy

© Parkinsons Recovery

Treatments for Tremors

- Take Medicine by Ear
- Vibrate Your Body
- Activate the Power of Your Mind
- Transform Beliefs that Inflame Tremors

I will now discuss some of the exciting options for each of approaches for calming tremors that are listed above. I suspect you will be fascinated by options you may well have never heard about.

You cannot do them all. As you preview the options, which ones "call out to you" to be further investigated? Which ones intrigue you? The options I discuss next have helped at least one person. May the next person it helps calm tremors be you!

Reduce Stress

Successful therapies for tremors focus on reducing stress. The idea is not to wrestle the tremor so that it becomes still. If you focus on "taming" your tremor as a lion tamer might go about taming a wild lion, the most likely outcome is that your tremor will become more rebellious. If you are serious about sedating tremors, you have to reduce your

24

stress level. Once the stress is under control, tremors can be calmed and sedated naturally.

Stress is a reality of life for everyone. Some days present more challenging symptoms (such as enhanced tremors) than other days. Research findings on stress are definitive. Stress is a primary cause of many illnesses and diseases including Parkinson's disease. It makes logical sense to have a tool kit of therapies that help reduce the moment to moment challenges of living in a stressful world.

How can this be accomplished? Reducing stress involves more than deciding to lead a "stress free" lifestyle. You have to work at it, but not so hard that you create even more stress frantically trying to get stress "under control." The methods I introduce next offer the opportunity to reduce your level of stress using very simple, effective techniques. You also have access to them any time of the day or night.

Triple Warmer
Meridians in the body connect to various organs and tissues. Knowledge of their existences has been known for centuries. Meridians are identified by such names as the

Treatments for Tremors

gall bladder meridian, the small intestine meridian, the stomach meridian, the large intestine meridian, the bladder meridian, the heart meridian and others. The name of the meridian identifies the affected organ.

Which meridian is responsible for tremoring? Several meridians are typically implicated, but tremors are fueled primarily by the "triple warmer" meridian. Never heard of it? Most people haven't unless they are acupuncturists.

Most illnesses in the physical body are caused by too little energy that runs through a meridian. The lack of flow is caused by an emotional or physical trauma to the body. In stark contrast, the triple warmer meridian stimulates tremors (and other conditions such as insomnia) when an excess of energy races through.

Are you often anxious? More specifically, are you anxious about the dangers that lurk throughout the world, the tenuous condition of your finances or the deteriorating health of yourself or family members? Are you even anxious about the potential risks of taking a leisurely stroll down the sidewalk of your neighborhood? If any of these possibilities resonate with you, your triple warmer meridian has an excess of energy rushing through it. The rapid flow needs to be reduced if tremors are to be sedated.

The ring finger on each hand is the termination point for the triple warmer meridian. Did your tremor originate in the ring finger of either hand or perhaps both hands? If so, there is a good possibility your triple warmer has been working on overdrive. An excess of energy has been gushing through your over-energized triple warmer meridian with the force of water flowing down Niagara Falls.

Why is reducing the flow of energy that races through the triple warmer meridian important for persons with tremors? Tremors will not be calmed until the energy running through your triple warmer meridian is reduced. Yes, more energy running through the body is usually desired. But, when the current of energy is excessive, the body cannot handle the load. Tremors are the consequence.

Electrical systems have transformers that stop the flow of electricity when it becomes over-charged. The body does not have a built in transformer to reduce or terminate the flow for a simple reason. If the flow is interrupted life can no longer exist. In a strange sense, tremors perform a function similar to that of transformers.

The body has a choice when an excessive charge of energy is confronted. It can either disperse the energy excess through tremoring of the hands, arms, legs or feet or it can contain the excess. The body always makes the rational decision to discharge the energy excess rather than contain it.

Consider the consequences if the excess is contained. Everyone knows that a healthy heart is critical to survival. Electrical impulses regulate heartbeats. If the electrical system in the body becomes overcharged, healthy function of the heart will be compromised. Containment of the excess flow of energy would endanger functionality of the heart in additional to all the other vital organs.

Instead of containing the excess energy, the body always chooses to disperse it through tremoring in an appendage (hands, arms, legs or feet). Tremors protect all the vital organs and the heart in particular from irrevocable harm.

Treatments for Tremors

The body places survival as its first priority. Tremors actually serve a function that can be critical to survival. When the excess of an energetic charge is dispersed through tremoring, a potentially life threatening meltdown (or heart attack) is averted.

Have you noticed that your tremors are more pronounced when you are stressed and/or emotions jettison out of control? The energy that is racing through your triple warmer meridian is overcharged. The excess sizzles through your nerve endings. Your nerves can't help but dance, rock, roll and gyrate all over the place. Of course the impact of the energy excess on your nerve endings is not experienced as a fun Saturday night dance. You are more familiar with the impact as a tremor that is strangely familiar, terribly annoying and painfully embarrassing. There is no doubt that tremors are a huge nuisance and embarrassment. The other side of the coin is that they also serve a critical purpose: they may be keeping you alive!

In addition to tremors do you also have insomnia? This is even more confirmation that you have an overactive triple warmer that begs to be sedated. The excess of energy

© Parkinsons Recovery

Treatments for Tremors

stimulates the adrenal glands to churn out an excess of adrenaline. The body is allocating its scarce resources to manufacture adrenaline. This is why you find yourself wide awake at night. The body is preoccupied with manufacturing adrenaline. It has no reserve of energy to make dopamine. You can't expect to have a restful sleep while riding as a passenger in an Indianapolis drag car race all night long.

You may well have already recognized the presence of an energy overflow that runs through your body and elected to reduce the overflow using one therapy or another. Prescription medications are a therapy of choice preferred by many people with Parkinson's. Have medications calmed your tremors? If so, yea! If not, consider other options.

One option I have to recommend is to reduce the rush of energy flowing through your triple warmer meridian. This therapy is free to do. You remain in control. And, it has no side effects as is the case with prescription medications. Before I explain this simple technique, I need to issue a warning.

Treatments for Tremors

The Triple Warmer Always Resists Sedation

The triple warmer does not like to be sedated! The therapy I am about to recommend must be done throughout the day when you are stressed. To experience long lasting results it should be practiced daily for at a minimum of 40 days without interruption.

I am now going to predict what will happen to you at the outset so you will not be surprised. You will do the triple warmer sedation therapy I describe below every day in the beginning - perhaps for 7 days, or 10 days or even 30 days. Then, guess what will happen? There will come a day out of the blue when you suddenly forget to do the therapy. On this day, you never even think about doing it - even though you have celebrated relief when you have been doing the therapy. In short, you will wind up abandoning the therapy. Worse, you will falsely convince yourself that this therapy is not helping to sedate your tremor.

I was given the same warning. As predicted, I forget to do my sedating exercise every day. Why does this happen? My only explanation for you is that the triple warmer has a consciousness all its own. I really do not have any better explanation for you other than – it happens.

© Parkinsons Recovery

Treatments for Tremors

When this does happen (if it does happen that is), simply start over. You will and can prevail. It may take several false starts. Don't let this discourage you. With clear intention, your will eventually persist for the full 40 days and will be in a position to access the technique when needed anywhere – anytime.

Sedate the Triple Warmer

The following technique for sedating your triple warmer meridian takes only 10-15 seconds. You probably thought I was going to suggest a technique that would take an hour or two, eh? The technique can be done repeatedly throughout the day. The more frequently you do it, the better the results. Be reminded to do this when your tremors are more troublesome.

You may experience an immediate result or not. The idea however is not to calm tremors immediately. The idea is to reduce the excessive flow of energy that is racing through your body. This is fueling a high intensity of stress that is riveting throughout your body. Tremors will settle down as the overall intensity and flow of energy running through your triple warmer is dispersed.

Treatments for Tremors

You obviously want a healthy current of energy running through this meridian, but not an excess. The goal is to siphon off the excess, not reduce the flow. The flow is your life force!

The mechanics of the technique I am about to explain are simple. It helps first to understand why this technique helps calm tremors. There is a starting point and an ending point to every meridian. If you want to increase the energy running through a meridian – in our case the triple warmer meridian - you need to increase the flow of energy running through it. The task at hand is to reduce the flow, not increase it. This is accomplished by running the energy through the meridian backwards. I realize this sounds complicated, but it is really easy to do.

The starting point of the triple warmer meridian is the ring finger (or fourth finger) at the base of the nail. The ending point of the meridian is a point on the outside edge of the eyebrow which is furthest from your nose. If you want to increase the energetic charge running through your triple warmer meridian, you would start with touching your ring finger and end with touching your eye brow. We want to sedate the energy. This means we must make a pass

© Parkinsons Recovery

Treatments for Tremors

through the meridian backwards – starting with touching the eye brow first and ending with touching the ring finger last.

Use the opposite hand to touch the outside edge of your eyebrow, furthest from your nose. In other words, use your right hand to touch your left eye brow.

Run your hand beginning from your eyebrow down to your ring finger as your circle your ear, touch down the back of your neck and across the back of your shoulder, then down the outside of your arm until you reach the back of your hand. End the circuit by touching your ring finger at the base of the nail.

Do this three times on each side. Use your left hand to touch your right eye brow to sedate the energy running through the right side of your body. Use your right hand to touch your left eye brow to sedate the energy running through the left side of your body.

If you want to know more about the precise details of where the triple warmer meridian runs through the body, do a quick search on the internet on the triple warmer. You will preview anatomy charts that show the precise flow of the triple warmer meridian line and its associated acupressure points.

The instructions above are simply tracking the meridian line from the end to the start. The critical steps are to touch eye brow first and the ring finger last. You can skip the scan down your neck, shoulder and arm and as a short cut simply touch the eye brow first and the ring finger second. Once you do one side three times, do the other three times. The exact path of your scan is not critical. You will need only to be sure and touch the exact start (eye brow) and end point (ring finger at the base of the nail).

The technique I am recommending is drawn from a therapy known as acupressure. A book you may want to borrow at the library or buy that I use as my primary resource is titled: *The Joy of Feeling: Body Mind Acupressure.*[7]

You can get very precise if you wish. There are precise contact points for this meridian along the neck, shoulder and arm. I think making the technique simple to do is best

---

[7]
http://www.amazon.com/gp/product/0870406345/ref=as_li_tl?ie=UT F8&camp=1789&creative=9325&creativeASIN=0870406345&linkCode =as2&tag=zerpoihea-20&linkId=3VGBQHUWRFXL6T43

myself. More importantly, sedating the triple warmer often will also help to calm it down and quiet tremors.

Sedate the Governing Vessel

Another point on the body that, when massaged, calms the nervous system and offers the opportunity to calm tremors is the end point of the Governing Vessel known as Acupuncture Point 20. This is the end point of a sequence of points in the Governing Vessel meridian that are spaced up and down your spine. You cannot massage many of the points along the spine because you cannot reach them. You can massage the most important point which happens to be located on the top of your head near the front.

Do not fret over the technical terms. Rather, watch this one minute video that demonstrates how to locate this point on the top of the head. This point is located in the middle of the head toward the front. As you will see demonstrated in this video[8], you will want to gently massage the point after you locate it on top of your head. Do this right now and experience the result.

---

[8] https://www.youtube.com/watch?v=i7JTy1bMqTs

Treatments for Tremors

What happened? Gently massaging this particular point releases the excess of energy that runs up the Governing Vessel meridian. Instead of being released through tremoring you can facilitate the release of the excess energy through another pathway – the top of the head.

The governing meridian helps maintain yin/yang balance or what is otherwise known as the male and female energies that reside within each of us. If there is an excess of energy racing through this meridian, male energy will overrun female energy. Female energy makes production of dopamine in the body possible. The idea behind gently massaging Acupuncture Point 20 of the Governing Vessel is to bring the male and female energies into balance.

Become Mindful

As noted previously, a sustained level of stress is the authentic troublemaker for tremors. Stress thunders through every cell of our bodies. It shatters nerves. The neurological system is profoundly affected. All systems of the body are jolted off balance.

When people experience stress, their tremors do get worse. When stress levels are under control, tremors subside. You see, the problem is not the tremor itself. The problem is stress. Tremors become manageable when stress becomes manageable.

A practical and powerful method for stress reduction is to embrace a dedicated practice of mindfulness. I fully realize that "mindfulness" is trendy and fashionable these days, but the underlying principles are sound.

Simply put, becoming more mindful means we are present in the moment rather than agonizing over a past that cannot be changed or worrying about a future that seldom materializes. A successful mindfulness practice means that we become totally and completely present to each and every moment of our lives. We live in the present moment without agonizing over the past or fretting about the future.

Stress exerts an unrelenting pressure on our bodies when we slip into the past with our thoughts or jump into the future with our worries. If we fixate on rehashing past experiences that were traumatic, hurtful or unpleasant – a rush of stress hormones are released. If we worry about what the future holds in store for us, we fixate on events that rarely happen anyway. When thoughts are centered in the past or future the body is suspended in a continual state of stress.

When the body is stressed, cells are flushed with blasts of adrenaline. This leaves little energy for the body to manufacture dopamine. Symptoms flourish under these conditions. We feed symptoms the perfect fertilizers: worry, fear, regret, guilt and anger.

Routine habits of worry, anxiety and stress have to be transformed. Our moment to moment thoughts must focus on the present and nowhere else. Simply put, becoming more mindful means that our thoughts, attention and energy focus on the present moment. A neurological system reset is required for most of us to become more mindful.

A successful practice of mindfulness – which does take practice – re-wires the neurological network. Becoming more mindful changes the worn out, embedded neurological pathways. Visualize these neurological pathways as deep ruts that were carved out by the pioneers traveling over the same roadways in covered wagons to the western states of the America.

Without a conscious mindfulness practice we fall back into the same habits of thinking that stimulate flushes of stress hormones. We persist in accessing the same neural pathways that excite tremors. Eventually, the neurological system freaks out. Recovery is dead ended. Transforming habits of thinking that are not in our best and highest good can be genuinely challenging. Put more directly, bad habits are hard to break!

Norman Doidge published a marvelous book titled *The Brain's Way of Healing*.[9] One chapter, "*A Man Walks Off his Parkinsonian Symptoms*" reports the story of a man from South Africa who used conscious control of his walking in combination with a vigorous pace (interrupted by rest). The result? He saw sustained relief from his

---

[9]

http://www.amazon.com/gp/product/067002550X/ref=as_li_tl?ie=UTF8&camp=1789&creative=9325&creativeASIN=067002550X&linkCode=as2&tag=zerpoihea-20&linkId=P3ZHHYPXZGHQLOPH

Treatments for Tremors

Parkinson's symptoms. Now, this is a form of mindfulness practiced the right way to be sure!

Recent research demonstrates that becoming mindful helps reverse Parkinson's symptoms. I do not personally have tremors or any of the symptoms of Parkinson's disease. But, when I discovered as a researcher the usefulness of mindfulness to health, I took stock of my own success with being mindful. I must confess that I flunked my own evaluation. I spent far more energy and time worrying about the future and fretting over the past than living in the present.

I created my own series of 52 challenges to support my intention to become more mindful. Then, I practiced each challenge for one full week over the course of a year.

- Practice did help me become more mindful.

- Practice did pave the way for my body to construct new neurological pathways.

I translated my discoveries into a series of mindfulness challenges that are issued each week for a year.[10] Each

© Parkinsons Recovery

challenge is accompanied by an explanation of its deeper implications for people who experience Parkinson's symptoms and tremors. Becoming more mindful gently releases tensions that assault the body and tug hormones out of whack.

For those who prefer paperbacks over emails, the mindfulness challenges were also organized into nine topics to help heighten awareness of how tension is held in the body. The Parkinsons Recovery Mindfulness series consists of nine paperbacks that cover the topics of seeing, hearing, noticing, doing, eating, thinking, feeling, being and intending. The challenges are also available as downloads.[11]

Let your intuition guide a choice as to how to practice mindfulness – whether that choice is to follow the program I have created or adopt another program. There are many excellent mindfulness programs that are now available. Of course, you can also design your own

---

[10] http://www.stress.parkinsonsrecovery.com

[11] http://www.parkinsonsrecovery.info

program which was my preference. The one most significant step you can take to sedate your tremors is to become more mindful however you decide to make that happen for yourself.

Hypnotize Yourself

Guess What? You do not have to employ a hypnotherapist to get hypnotized. You can make it happen all by yourself! Hypnotherapist Steve Frison offered a fascinating presentation at the Vancouver Parkinsons Recovery Summit when he discussed the use of hypnotherapy as an adjunct therapy for Parkinson's. He taught self-hypnosis techniques to Summit participants that help people improve relaxation and reduce stress. Steve has a rich variety of resources that are available on his website.[12]

Steve argues that hypnotherapy can help you...

- Reaffirm that you are not your diagnosis.
- Improve mental acuity and decision making.
- Feel more passionate, joyous and motivated about life.

---

[12] http://www.mindsighthypno.com/trauma-hypnosis.html

Treatments for Tremors

- Move freely and easily with confidence and comfort.
- Remember how you moved your body before the onset of Parkinson's symptoms.
- Improve the depth and quality of sleep.
- Reduce and relax muscles.
- Balance and return neurotransmitters to optimal levels.
- Strengthen your immune system.
- Improve the body's ability to differentiate the body's healthy cells from viruses, bacteria and abnormal cells (which are also alive).

Move Your Body Gently

Researcher and clinician Richard Brown MD has extensive experience working with individuals with Parkinson's symptoms. One of his strongest recommendations for people with tremors and other symptoms of Parkinson's disease is to move their body slowly and gently using the ancient systems of Tai Chi or QiGong.

© Parkinsons Recovery

Treatments for Tremors

Tai Chi

Practiced for thousands of years in the East, Tai Chi involves relatively slow, repetitive movements that help bring the body back into balance and harmony. It helps focus the mind solely on the form of the movements. This brings about a state of mental calm and 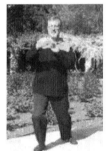 clarity. It is a delicious therapy that you can incorporate into your exercise routine every day.

Daniel Loney was one of my early guests on the Parkinsons Recovery Radio show[13] who alerted me to the enormous benefits of Tai Chi:

> *"I could continue running around and spending lots of money looking for a cure or take responsibility for my own health and get on with it. I already possessed the necessary tools for dealing with Parkinson's. They had been there from the beginning.*

Daniel had practiced Tai Chi before his diagnosis of Parkinson's disease, but set his commitment to Tai Chi

---

[13] http://www.blogtalkradio.com/parkinsons-recovery/2009/12/03/pioneers-of-recovery

© Parkinsons Recovery

aside when his Parkinson's symptoms became problematic. His teacher, Arieh Breslow was also a guest on the Parkinsons Recovery radio show.[14] After reinvigorating his personal practice of Tai Chi, Danny's tremors became virtually nonexistent.

Recent research has shown impressive benefits for people with Parkinson's symptoms who practice Tai Chi. It would have died out thousands of years ago had it not provided compelling benefits to millions of people. It really did not take a multi-million dollar research study for anyone to realize that Tai Chi clears the energetic cobwebs that obstruct the intention to heal and flushes the toxins that are embedded in your tissues and organs.

Daniel Loney[15] has an eloquent explanation of why Tai Chi helps reduce Parkinson's symptoms:

> Tai Chi is an internal martial art form that uses the mind to control the movements of the body. It helps you become aware of your body and the integration of each part with the whole. Visual

---

[14] http://www.blogtalkradio.com/parkinsons-recovery/2009/08/06/pioneers-of-recovery
[15] http://www.taichiparkinsons.com

imagery is used to help in this mind–body connection and to aid in movement and coordination. The slow, deliberate movements of the Tai Chi form can directly address many of the major Parkinson's symptoms.

QiGong

A companion modality to Tai Chi is QiGong, Bianca Molle[16] found QiGong to be a godsend for her. She writes that:

> *"The worst tremor was in my left hand and I am left-handed. I also had tremor activity on the right side."*

She reversed these symptoms along with other troubling

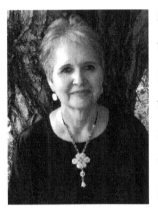

symptoms of Parkinson's disease with a focused and dedicated practice of QiGong. Do not expect to attend a one day QiGong retreat and expect your tremors will vanish. Results do happen for people with Parkinson's symptoms when they commit to a daily QiGong practice.

---

[16] http://www.mettamorphix.com

© Parkinsons Recovery

Treatments for Tremors

Bianca offers an eloquent explanation for the theory behind QiGong:

> *"The ancient Chinese believed that almost all disease was caused by a blockage of energy. The theory is that illness will disappear by getting energy to move through the body freely. Ninety-six percent (96%) of the energy in the universe is unseen. We see only 4% from our contact with the physical world. Qigong practice invokes this unseen energy. The different movements of Qigong practice and the different meditations of the practice direct the energy to where it needs to go to heal the body. Chi energy also has its own intelligence. Sometimes it naturally goes to places on its own that need to be healed."*

If QiGong calls out to you as a therapy to calm your stress and relieve your anxiety, I recommend that you investigate several additional resources. My Parkinsons Recovery radio show[17] interview with Bianca has been transcribed and is now available as a paperback from Amazon.[18]

[17] http://www.blogtalkradio.com/parkinsons-recovery/2011/06/15/metamorphesis-shakin-to-awaken

Treatments for Tremors

Alternatively, I invite you to listen to my radio show interview with Bianca that was recorded, archived and is readily accessible. This is one of the many free services I offer through Parkinsons Recovery.

The second radio program[19] is an interview with my guest Bill Bulick who, like Bianca, also found QiGong to be a solution to calming his Parkinson's symptoms. And also just like Bianca, Bill has a deep understanding of what it really takes to heal from the inside out.

FeldenKrais

Irene Pasternack[20] demonstrates how tremors can be reduced through an enhanced understanding of the structure of the arm and shoulders which are affected most directly when we are stressed. People who took advantage of her free sessions and classes during the

---

18
http://www.amazon.com/gp/product/1502981661/ref=as_li_tl?ie=UT F8&camp=1789&creative=9325&creativeASIN=1502981661&linkCode =as2&tag=zerpoihea-20&linkId=RMVHFV4GBXUE6GHM

19 http://www.blogtalkradio.com/parkinsons-recovery/2015/05/18/qigong-for-health-and-happiness-workshop-1

20
http://www.movebeyondlimits.com/Parkinsons_and_Feldenkrais.htm

Treatments for Tremors

Parkinsons Recovery Vancouver Summit said that they found Feldenkrais™ to be an extremely useful therapy.

Want to become more knowledgeable about how Feldenkrais™ helps people with tremors? Watch the video that is posted on the Parkinsons Recovery blog.[21]

Release Trauma

Trauma gets embedded at the cellular level. The Chinese have known for centuries that energy (or chi) that should naturally flow through the meridians of the body often gets clogged, twisted and obstructed. Visualize driving down a highway that is under repair. Numerous detours are required. Travel on gravel road surfaces takes its own toll on the life of your tires. Various therapies help to repave the roadways and remove the detours so that the energy flows freely through the meridians without being distorted, side tracked or dammed up.

Many people with tremors experience an unrelenting feeling of anxiousness and fear. Trauma lies at the

---

[21] http://www.blog.parkinsonsrecovery.com/how-to-reduce-tremors-naturally

Treatments for Tremors

foundation of nervousness that spins out of control. The key to calming the excitation is to release the trauma that is trapped at the cellular level. The consciousness of traumas is literally glued to the tissues until they are detached and purged.

Most people I know hold onto traumas their entire lifetime. They assume the continuing pain and suffering from traumas that were experienced at a time long ago and at a place far away must be tolerated and endured. This is one of those false beliefs that have never been true. Set the intention to release any and all trauma and it will be done.

A Word of Caution about Trauma Releases

Before I preview the options for you to consider I have a word of caution about trauma releases. If you are like me, you will be driven to purge all traces of trauma right now! Why wait I say and you may be saying the same thing.

The problem with this attitude is that the body can gyrate all over the place during releases. The process of releasing trauma (regardless of the method employed) can exhaust the physical body as it may need to shake, twist and flop all over the place for the release to take full effect. When the trauma begins to "blow out", it is often helpful to have a skilled therapist present so you do not hurt yourself!

It may feel weird during releases. You may become very tired. But, trust me on this - after a few days you will feel lighter and more energetic. When you experience a release using any therapy, give your body at least a 3-4 day (and preferably a week) break to recover.

When it feels like enough toxic residue from past traumas has been released, stop! You can continue the release at a later time. With a little experimentation you will discover approaches and methods for releasing trauma that work beautifully for you. Your body (and you) will like some of the suggestions I have for you and perhaps not like other suggestions. Do not expect all of the traumas that are trapped in your physical body to flood out in one session or even using one therapy. Traumas are not purged with a single treatment. Rather, releasing trauma is a lifetime process.

Treatments for Tremors

Everyone has trauma that has been trapped in the tissues of their body. People who do not succeed in releasing traumas will eventually get sick.

Releases of trauma from the physical and energetic body dismantle the blockages that have been obstructing recovery. Once the obstructions have been cleared and the dark energy released, the body gets down to the creative work of healing those highly sensitive and very juicy neural pathways.

The character of trapped trauma is heavy. It drains our enthusiasm for life and exhausts our energy. The markers of trauma are usually buried deep inside our tissues. With each release, a deeper layer can be accessed and released. It is exciting work because it helps you feel so much better! Over time, I predict that you will celebrate one victory after another as your tremors become less problematic.

What follows are some possibilities to consider. They all do work wonders, but only one or perhaps several will be the best strategy for you to pursue.

Treatments for Tremors

Most people think of mediation as a therapy that involves only one technique: Sit with your legs crossed and blank out all thoughts. Some people find this approach to meditation to be valuable. Others experience even more stress.

The release meditation I recommend involves a structured approach that identifies, corrals and releases traumas that have been stored and embedded in your cells for years, if not decades.

Doing the release meditation on a regular basis has proved very beneficial and very powerful to me personally as well as to many others. Once you learn the "release meditation template," it is easy to use and takes 10 minutes (or longer if you choose). You are in control when doing the release meditation. Your own thoughts do not have any chance of kidnapping your intention to reduce stress.

Since we are all re-traumatized by one experience or another, you have to continue doing the release mediation. Otherwise, new traumas will stifle your energy and clog up your energy pathways. Do this meditation when you feel stressed and overwhelmed. It will help you feel much lighter and better overall. It costs nothing. Best of all, it always puts you in the driver's seat.

When trauma remains trapped in our body, the chances for calming tremors are slim. When we succeed with releasing past and current traumas, chances for recovery skyrocket.

A video of the release meditation I use every week and recommend to others for releasing trauma can be watched by visiting the website referenced in this footnote.[22] This demonstration of the release meditation was taped at the Parkinsons Recovery Summit in Santa Fe, New Mexico USA.

Emotional Freedom Technique

Emotional Freedom Technique (EFT) is a tapping technique some people use to release trauma. I personally do not place it in the same category as acupuncture which, as you know, is a therapy that involves a licensed acupuncturist who inserts needles in your body. Acupuncture can facilitate the release of trauma, but you give up control.

[22] http://www.healing.summit.parkinsonsrecovery.com

Treatments for Tremors

With EFT, you remain in full control with regard to how you do it, when you do it and where you do it. Someone else is not making these decisions for you.

From the research on EFT I have seen, it is safe and noninvasive. You can always administrator EFT to yourself. It is a gentle, simple way to re-program the energy pathways in the body.

There is an excellent resource that provides a free, comprehensive tutorial on EFT offered by Gary Craig, a founder of EFT. Be sure to watch the 7 minute video on the main page of his website referenced in this footnote[23]. The video offers an excellent overview of EFT. On the top menu of this web site there are links to pages that provide detailed instruction on how you can learn EFT.

Look over the free training information and see what you think. The website also offers certifications for EFT practitioners, but you do not have to be certified to practice EFT on yourself every day. EFT is a therapy you

---

[23] http://www.emofree.com

© Parkinsons Recovery

can practice right now that offers the possibility of relief from your tremors. Why not give it a spin? It is free.

There is an amazing video referenced in this footnote[24] of war veterans who used EFT. Watching this video will inspire you learn more about EFT. The downside is that it lasts 20 minutes to watch from the beginning to end but it is well worth taking the time to watch. The video previews the benefit of EFT for war veterans who have PTSD (Post Traumatic Stress Syndrome). It does not focus specifically on people with tremors or those who have been diagnosed with Parkinson's disease. When you watch the video, you will see many of the war veterans have tremors. Why? They were traumatized by their experiences in combat when serving in Vietnam, Iraq or elsewhere.

Everyone responds differently to any therapy to calm tremors. EFT may not succeed in calming your tremors. Then again, it may work miracles! EFT has been around for quite a while and has grown in acceptance every year

---

[24] https://www.youtube.com/watch?v=B4hhMm8qsCs

because, I think, it is safe and easy to do anytime of the day or night. I have personally never known anyone who has had a negative experience with EFT, though not everyone experiences the outcome they hoped for.

In the end, use your intuition and gut instincts to decide whether to learn more about EFT. If it feels right, give it a try. You can probably tell if it helps to calm your tremors relatively quickly. If it does not feel right, look elsewhere. I am now sounding like a broken record, but always take charge of your recovery decisions!

Breathwork

Breathwork is a therapy that uses continuous breathing in and out without pausing. Breathwork facilitates release of emotions that were frozen from traumatic experiences. It removes trapped emotions by literally lifting them out of your physical body. Deep emotions will surface – some of them unpleasant. Some people find it is useful to limit each session to only a minute or two or to a limited number of breaths in and out.

To learn more about why therapy can be so beneficial, take a minute right now to do continuous breathing for a minute or two. Emotions do surface. This brief experience will help you better understand why Breathwork can be beneficial to releasing trauma.

What is the rationale for using Breathwork to release trauma? If we breathe when we are traumatized, the unpleasant emotions are released. But, we usually do not breathe when confronted with traumatic situations. No. We stop breathing. It is the best way to kill unpleasant emotions.

The strategy to stop breathing works beautifully to kill unpleasant emotions. Great I say. It works for me. The unfortunate consequence of this strategy is the effects of trauma are trapped in the physical body rather than being released. Trapped trauma causes tremors.

To summarize, emotions are released when we breathe deeply. Breathwork releases the effects of trauma that has been trapped in our bodies through deep, continuous breathing.[25] Trained and certified therapists are available

---

[25] http://www.takingcharge.csh.umn.edu/explore-healing-practices/breathwork

[26] http://www.goodtherapy.org/breathwork.html#

in most localities who can extend hands on assistance using the method.[26] Or, you can begin doing Breathwork today without the assistance of a trained facilitator and see where it takes you. Either way, keep the end goal in mind: Release the trauma to calm the tremors.

Energy Healing

Illness in the physical body arises out of distortions in the human energy field. The originating cause for tremors will be evident in the energy field (which can be detected by energy healers) long before they are experienced as tremors.

Most people devote their attention to treating the tremors as a physical imbalance. Since the reason for the tremor originated in the human energy field – it is actually more expedient (and less expensive) to repair distortions in the human energy field. The more efficient way to calm tremors down is not to engage a frontal attack on the physical body itself. Rather, the approach that promises far greater success in the long run is to clear distortions in the energy field.

Treatments for Tremors

The distortions themselves can take many forms including holes and tears in the energy field. Experienced energy healers have the training to detect and address these problems. Removing obstructions and clearing blockages in the energy field are necessary for tremors to be quieted permanently.

Brennan Healing Science is one among a variety of "energy healing" therapies that bring a distorted, contorted energy field back into balance and harmony. The approach combines hands-on healing techniques with spiritual and psychological support.

There is a comprehensive listing of graduates on the Barbara Brennan website. Graduates are located in most cities and countries throughout the world. Click on the "Find a Practitioner" link to locate a graduate of the four year program who practices in your city.[27]

I attended the Barbara Brennan School of Healing as a student for four years after experiencing the unexpected death of my wife Nanette. Her untimely death was a trauma I was unable to get over without assistance. I

[27] http://www.barbarabrennan.com

found the experience at the school to be enlightening and useful. I am certainly not recommending that you enroll as a student. I do recommend that you contact graduates from your locality listed on the Barbara Brennan website to discuss the possibility of an appointment.

A companion "energy healing" modality you may have heard about is Reiki. Sunday Connections host Karl Robb[28] and his wife Angela are Reiki healers. Karl, the author of *A Soft Voice in a Noisy World: A Guide to Dealing and Healing with Parkinson's Disease*[29] has found Reiki to be a therapy that helps reverse his own Parkinson's symptoms.

Do not expect one appointment with an energy healer to work miracles. Healing from the inside-out is a journey. Once the traumas have been released, other underlying reasons for tremors can be addressed. Energy healing will help to release any and all traumas that sustain symptoms like tremors. Of course, energy healing treatments can also facilitate healing of symptoms other than tremors.

---

[28] https://pdpatient.wordpress.com
[29]
http://www.amazon.com/gp/product/0988184702/ref=as_li_tl?ie=UTF8&camp=1789&creative=9325&creativeASIN=0988184702&linkCode=as2&tag=zerpoihea-20

Treatments for Tremors

Bowen Therapy

Bowen Therapy[30] was originally developed in Australia.

The Bowen practitioner:

- Moves, positions and holds hands, feet, arms or legs in various positions for releases.
- Gently rolls the body or positions the body for releases.
- Focuses on the release of trauma and tension throughout the entire body.

Craniosacral Therapy

Craniosacral Therapy[31] is gentle. Touch is equivalent to the weight of a dime resting on the body.

- The therapist exerts pressure that is no greater than the weight of a dime.
- The therapist works on or off the body.
- Focus is on cranial sacral system – the system that comprises the brain, spine and sacrum.

---

[30] http://www.nsthealth.com/practitioners

[31] http://www.iahp.com/pages/search/index.php

© Parkinsons Recovery

Treatments for Tremors

The Emotion Code

Bradley Nelson developed a method of finding and releasing specific "trapped emotions," a term he assigns to emotions that are literally "stuck" in the body. He has written a book titled *The Emotion Code*[32] which outlines the method. Many people learn the method from instructions on the internet or from reading his book. The method can be done by yourself or using a trained practitioner.

Trapped Emotions stick to the tissues in the body from the time we were conceived. Or, they can be literally inherited from ancestors who lived at a time far away and long ago. The average person has many emotions that are trapped. Those with chronic illness have many more.

Many doctors believe that most health issues are tied to emotional stress. Dr. Nelson believes that the persistent stress from trapped emotions is responsible for over 50% of pain. In his book, he writes: "I have seen hundreds of

---

[32]

http://www.amazon.com/gp/product/0979553709/ref=as_li_tl?ie=UTF8&camp=1789&creative=9325&creativeASIN=0979553709&linkCode=as2&tag=zerpoihea-20&linkId=A7R6VPXYERPJRWAS

cases where acute physical pain instantly left the body upon the release of a trapped emotion."

A marvelous resource who does long distance Emotion Code consultations is John O'Dwyer. His wife was diagnosed with Parkinson's disease. John is a valuable resource who helps people release traumas using the Emotion Code as well as other trauma release therapies.[33]

Myofascial Release

The intention behind Myofascial Release is to relax muscles that have contracted and stiffened and, in so doing, improve circulation of blood and lymph. The work untangles restrictions in the fascia which become entangled from trauma. Fascia is found throughout the body. It is a thin, tough, elastic tissue that wraps around tissues and muscles. Fascia supports and protects these structures.

Physical Therapist David Howell presented an excellent explanation of myofascial release on the Parkinsons Recovery Radio Show.[34] Listen to the program where he

---

[33] http://www.chichoices.com

[34] http://www.blogtalkradio.com/parkinsons-

offers an eloquent explanation of this therapeutic approach to releasing trauma that is trapped at the cellular level.

Take Supplements and Herbs

The Chinese view Parkinson's symptoms as a liver-wind deficiency. People shake or tremor who have this deficiency. A more straightforward way to explain this deficiency is:

- The liver is toxic.
- The kidneys are functioning considerably below capacity.

Sedation of tremors requires that you purge toxins from the liver and improve the functionality of your kidneys. It is more important to get the bad stuff out of your body before putting the good stuff in – which is the first of the *Seven Secrets to Healing*.[35] Be circumspect in whatever choices you make about taking any of the supplements I

---

recovery/2010/04/15/pioneers-of-recovery
[35]
http://www.amazon.com/gp/product/1497423287/ref=as_li_tl?ie=UTF8&camp=1789&creative=9325&creativeASIN=1497423287&linkCode=as2&tag=zerpoihea-20&linkId=NAVMTBPALN46OG7C

will recommend to calm tremors. Yes, they may indeed help. In the long run, priority needs to be placed on getting toxins out of the organs in your body – and the liver in particular – first. My personal experience with healing[36] is that toxins are an issue for everyone – not just persons with tremors.

Supplements and herbs are discussed next that potentially have a beneficial impact on quieting tremors. They are natural substances that can be acquired without a prescription from a doctor. These supplements and herbs are still medicines however. Side effects tend to be less problematic than prescription medicines, but you may still incur side effects. Be sure to consult with your doctor and/or pharmacist before taking any of the supplements or herbs that are suggested next. They may possibly interact or interfere with prescription medications your doctor has already prescribed.

---

[36]
http://www.amazon.com/gp/product/1508516812/ref=as_li_tl?ie=UTF8&camp=1789&creative=9325&creativeASIN=1508516812&linkCode=as2&tag=zerpoihea-20&linkId=JTT5GOGU4AEDNF4M

Treatments for Tremors

Mucuna?

Medical doctors prescribe medications to supplement L-Dopa which the body needs to make dopamine. Since all medications have side effects, some people prefer to take alternatives to the prescription medications that do not have the documented side effects of medications. One such substance is the herb Mucuna which, incidentally, is also a medication. You just do not need a prescription from a medical doctor to get it. There is a form of Mucuna that does require a prescription, but it is very expensive to acquire.

I have heard scattered reports on the effectiveness of Mucuna to calm tremors. Some people praise its effectiveness. Others report it had little or no effect. Why in the world do the reports vary so widely?

I believe the reason for the vastly different experiences people report is the quality of the source. Most Mucuna is grown commercially. Its quality, or "energetic charge", is minimal. In other words, you are paying a lot of money for a minimal result.

© Parkinsons Recovery

Treatments for Tremors

I was quite surprised that Mucuna was not even mentioned in my interview with a highly qualified herbalist, Andrew Bentley. Why doesn't Andrew recommend Mucuna to his patients who have tremors? The answer surprised me. He had been unable to find a reliable, high quality supply of Mucuna. He buys other herbs he cannot grow himself in Kentucky from countries across the globe but has never been successful in finding a reliable source for Mucuna. Andrew recommends his patients take herbs for tremors other than Mucuna.

If I knew of a source that I could confidently recommend, I certainly would include here in a footnote, but I have none to recommend. I do have another recommendation for you to consider – the supplement NADH.

NADH

I do recommend that you talk with your doctor about taking NADH as a supplement. It can be acquired at any health food store without a prescription. There are so many supplements that could be taken, why do I suggest you consider taking NADH?

Treatments for Tremors

Tremors are associated with a deficiency of L-Dopa, a substance the body needs in sufficient quantity to manufacture dopamine. When you take a prescription medication like Sinemet or a herb like Mucuna or a food like fava beans, you are giving your body an extra hit of L-Dopa.

OK. So good so far. How is L-Dopa manufactured by the body? It uses Tyrosine, a natural substance in everyone's body, to make L-Dopa. This is why some people with tremors take Tyrosine as one of their supplements. It would seem to make logical sense to simply take more Tyrosine? Right? Unfortunately many people who take Tyrosine still have a tremor. So, why doesn't taking Tyrosine quiet their tremors?

Well, taking Tyrosine may be a good strategy for you. I have a quite different recommendation that was inspired by my radio show interview[37] with Compounding Pharmacist Randy Mentzer. The problem may not be a deficiency of Tyrosine, but the inability of the body to convert Tyrosine into L-Dopa. Randy explains that NADH is

---

[37] http://www.blogtalkradio.com/parkinsons-recovery/2009/11/25/pioneers-of-recovery

the substance that is used by the body to convert Tyrosine into L-Dopa. The body may not be able to convert Tyrosine into L-dopa – not because there is a deficiency of Tyrosine – but because there is a deficiency of NADH. Randy recommends that people talk with their doctors about taking NADH as a supplement. More than a "normal" dose may be needed in the short run to kick start the conversion process.

Randy Mentzer is not the only expert who recommends taking NADH. Steven Fowkes conducted two decades of research on Parkinson's and offered a number of suggestions during my interview with him for any and all persons searching for ways to find relief from their symptoms. As you will learn from listening to my interview with him on **Parkinsons Recovery Radio**[38], Steve Fowkes says that approximately 40% of the individuals who currently experience the symptoms of Parkinson's have a NADH deficiency. He, like Randy, also recommends that anyone currently experiencing the symptoms of Parkinson's like tremors consider taking NADH. Why not take it and see if you experience an improvement in your

---

[38] http://www.blogtalkradio.com/parkinsons-recovery/2009/06/11/pioneers-of-recovery

Treatments for Tremors

tremor? Maybe you will fall in that 40% minority who do experience a positive outcome. According to Steven Fowkes (as you will hear in the interview), taking NADA can't do any harm and offers a reasonable chance of getting at least some relief from tremors.

Glutathione

Research on Parkinson's reveals a pattern. The brain has far too many free radicals. This is what causes cellular damage. An overabundance of free radicals in the brain is one cause (but not necessarily the only cause) of tremors.

How do you extinguish this "raging fire" of too many free radicals that are having a 24 hour a day party in your brain? Any anti-oxidant should provide some relief – and there are many – but the brain has a preferred antioxidant. It is called Glutathione.

The solution to tremors would seem obvious at this point. Simply pour more Glutathione into the brain. The glitch with this seemingly smart idea is that little (if any) glutathione taken orally actually reaches the brain. It is poorly absorbed by the intestines and struggles to pass through the blood brain barrier. Taking Glutathione as an

© Parkinsons Recovery

oral supplement is considered by most health care professional as a waste of money.

Some doctors give Glutathione IV injections to their patients. This can be beneficial, but it is problematic for several reasons. First, getting Glutathione injections is costly. Second, many doctors recommend IV treatments three times a week. This means you have to travel to the doctor's office on three separate days each week. What a drag! Worse, how much stress can a person tolerate?

There is an alternative that Dr. Laurie Mischley ND prescribes for her patients with considerable success. She recommends use of a nasal Glutathione applicator. Talk with your doctor about the possibility of getting a prescription for the Glutathione nasal applicator. It is much less expensive than IV injections and requires no visits to the doctor's office. You only have to remember to spray the Glutathione up your nose several times a day.

Listen to my back to back radio show interviews[39] with Dr. Mischley to learn more about the Glutathione nasal

---

[39] http://www.blogtalkradio.com/parkinsons-recovery/2010/06/24/natural-therapies-for-parkinsons-disease

http://www.blogtalkradio.com/parkinsons-recovery/2010/07/01/the-option. Her book, *Natural Therapies for Parkinson's Disease*[40], is worth purchasing. It is a genuine treasure. The information she provides is worth all the gold in Fort Knox, Kentucky for anyone who experiences Parkinson's symptoms. A high quality glutathione nasal spray (available only with a doctor's prescription) can be purchased through Key Compounding Pharmacy[41] in Washington state once you get a prescription from your doctor.

CoQ10

People with the symptoms of Parkinson's have insufficient ATP (Adenosine triphosphate). Some studies find that individuals with Parkinson's have a 44% reduction in symptoms when they take a CoQ10 supplement. This is why doctors recommend that their patients take it.

---

most-important-step-you-can-take-to-recover

40

http://www.amazon.com/gp/product/1603810439/ref=as_li_tl?ie=UTF8&camp=1789&creative=9325&creativeASIN=1603810439&linkCode=as2&tag=zerpoihea-20&linkId=VEPP432XQWN5RQ6H

[41] http://www.keycompounding.com

Treatments for Tremors

CoQ10 plays a central role in helping the body generate energy in the form of ATP. Over 90% of the body's energy is generated this way. Organs with the highest energy requirements—such as the heart and the liver—have the highest CoQ10 concentrations. Cardiologists often recommend CoQ10 to their patients.

It is not unusual to hear someone diagnosed with Parkinson's disease say:

> *"I tried CoQ10 and it did nothing for me."*

You may have heard this report as well. Some research studies have also reported disappointing results. CoQ10 is a fundamental building block of the body, so logically speaking, it should make a big difference. There is a reason who some people experience disappointing results and research studies are unenthusiastic.

It is an expensive supplement which can potentially cost hundreds of dollars a month. Understandably, most people want to save money whenever possible, so they shop around for the best price on CoQ10 possible. I realize this is a strong statement, but I now believe that if you are not willing to pay for a high quality CoQ10 – do not even bother.

Treatments for Tremors

- *You are wasting your money.*
- *You are taking a substance that is toxic to your body because it cannot absorb it. It just has to turn around get rid of it.*
- *You wind up asking your kidneys to work overtime.*
- *You are adding waste that your liver has to process.*

In other words, you are throwing the money you spent down the toilet – literally.

If you decide your body needs CoQ10, get the highest quality available. Dr. Mischley[42] ND recommends two high quality sources of CoQ10: Vitaline and Douglas Labs which offers a wafer version of CoQ10 which they call Q Melt. Many health food stores carry these brands.

Sam-E

People who experience Parkinson's symptoms are low in S-adenosylmethinone – otherwise known as Sam-E. There is a logical reason for this widespread deficiency. Levodopa depletes Sam-E in the body relatively quickly. Sam-E is

---

[42]

http://www.amazon.com/gp/product/1603810439/ref=as_li_tl?ie=UTF8&camp=1789&creative=9325&creativeASIN=1603810439&linkCode=as2&tag=zerpoihea-20&linkId=6PE2IPPBG77U2RBL

responsible for a multitude of essential functions in the body which include boosting levels of glutathione. It is a protective agent for a liver that has been inundated with too many toxins.

What functions does Sam-E perform in the body? It:

- *Boosts high energy molecules*
- *Protects the body against harmful effects of stress*
- *Recharges the neurological system*
- *Sharpens mental clarity*
- *Enhances concentration*
- *Holds attention to tasks*
- *Heightens pleasure*
- *Serves as a natural anti-depressant*
- *Improves mood*
- *Heals nerve cell membranes*

For more information about the beneficial effects of Sam-E on alleviating many of the symptoms associated with Parkinson's including tremors, listen to my fascinating radio show interview with Richard Brown, MD who is the leading expert on its beneficial effects for Parkinson's disease.[43]

Treatments for Tremors

Magnesium Lotion

Most people these days have a magnesium deficiency.
Why? Most of us do not get sufficient magnesium in the
food that we eat. Magnesium plays a central role in
facilitating electrical cell signaling in the body. Tremors can
be the unfortunate consequence for persons with a
magnesium deficiency.

Magnesium plays a central role in facilitating more than
300 chemical reactions in the body. Potassium regulates
nerve functions. The body has to have sufficient
magnesium to transport the potassium to the cellular
membranes. In short, a deficiency of magnesium obstructs
the delivery of potassium to the cells, resulting in
neurological disturbances that manifest in the body as
tremors in the hands, feet or elsewhere.

In summary, magnesium helps to reduce tremors. It can
also facilitate a detoxing of heavy metals and other
harmful toxins which contribute to the neurological
challenge of tremors.

---

[43] http://www.blogtalkradio.com/parkinsons-
recovery/2013/07/24/integrative-and-complementary-treatments-for-
parkinsons

Treatments for Tremors

Some people have the mistaken idea that if they have a deficiency of one type or another (such as magnesium) they have to take a supplement or medicine by mouth. The skin is the largest organ in the body. I believe that magnesium deficiencies can more efficiently be addressed by applying a magnesium lotion on the skin. I personally apply Ancient Minerals Magnesium[44] lotion to my feet, legs and arms every day after I shower. You can take a magnesium supplement by mouth, but I think the better choice is to apply the lotion.

Herbs

Herbs are medicines too. They just usually have fewer side effects (or no side effects) and do not require a prescription. The particular form of herb that has the potential to sedate tremors depends on a variety of factors. Every person's situation is unique. It would be sweet if the answer would be "Take herb X and you are sure to see relief." The neurological system is far more complicated than most people realize.

---

[44] http://www.ancient-minerals.com

Treatments for Tremors

Andrew Bentley[45], a highly talented herbalist from Lexington, Kentucky who is an adjunct teacher at the University of Kentucky Medical School suggests several herbs that can potentially address problems with tremors. The particular herb or herbs that may successfully treat your tremor depend on a variety of factors including your body type and overall metabolic constitution.

If someone has a lot of tremors but no pain, Andrew Bentley says that:

> *"A herb that is an anti-spasmodic might help more than if someone is experiencing a lot of pain and rigidity, in which case we might use an entirely separate type of thing. Some things are helpful more or less across the board."*

Andrew reported that some of his patients with Parkinson's symptoms report that use of herbs such as Barley Malt Extract, Oat Straw, Valerian and Passion Flower have offered tremor relief. Whether any of these

---

[45] http://www.kentucky.com/2011/11/08/1950502/lexington-herbalist-offers-individualized.html

herbs can actually help you will depend on the level of dopamine in your body and whether or not the dopamine that is present is currently being absorbed.

Again, herbs are just as much a medicine as a prescription medicine. It is important to consult with your doctor when supplementing any prescription medicine with herbal medicines. Taking any herbal medicine that has the direct or indirect effect of bolstering dopamine levels will influence the dose and effectiveness of whatever prescription medications you might now be taking.

Barley Malt Extract

Barley Malt Extract is probably one herb you have never heard of, but Andrew reports it can potentially help with increasing levels of dopamine in the brain. The malt in barley extract comes from barley that has been sprouted and then concentrated into a soluble fiber. It has similar properties to other soluble fibers such as psyllium (Metamucil), oats and pectin in fruits. It creates better stool bulk and promotes bowel regularity. Beneficial bacteria in the colon use this fiber for food.

The Barley malt mixture does contain calories, so if you are trying to gain weight, this might be an option to consider

Treatments for Tremors

(though weight gain is rarely an issue for persons who currently experience tremors).

Oat Straw

Oat straw[46] can also be helpful for tremors. A lot of herbs that have anti-spasmodic effects also cause sedation. Andrew explains that oat straw usually does not cause drowsiness.

The oat straw (dried stems) and the grain are recommended for the treatment of a wide range of nervous conditions. The plant has also been shown to help with exhaustion from neurological pains and insomnia.

Oat straw contains protein (gluten), saponins, flavonoids, alkaloids, steroidal compounds, vitamins B1, B2, D, E, carotene, starch and fat. It also contains minerals such as calcium, magnesium and iron and trace elements like silicon and potassium.

---

[46] http://www.herbal-supplement-resource.com/oat-straw.html

Treatments for Tremors

Valerian

Andrew Bentley explains that :

> "Valerian is a much stronger herb for helping to suppress tremors but it does carry some risk of sedation, of feeling more drowsy and so forth especially when people first start taking it. Sometimes that lessons as time goes on. It is a very strong substance when it comes to helping control involuntary muscle movement tremors and involuntary movement of otherwise involuntary muscles. It is a good one for that.

Passion Flower

Andrew also suggests Passion Flower as a possibility for tremors:

> "Passion flower is also one that is helpful for some particular individuals. These are all things that would go into that category of working on tremors.

© Parkinsons Recovery

Treatments for Tremors

Ashwagandha

The herb Ashwagandha has been identified in research as a useful remedy for tremors, freezing and muscle pain.

One of the best, natural sources of dopamine can be found in not just herbs but certain foods. I introduce some exciting possibilities next.

Eat Wisely

Most people want to know what they can put into their body that promises the greatest chance of relief from tremors. Eliminating certain foods from your diet has the potential to offer greater returns – far greater than anything you cram into your body however "natural" or "organic" it might be.

One of the most dangerous toxins you can ingest is sugar. If you are dead serious about sedating your tremor, you must make the decision to stop putting sugar into your body. Sticking to this decision is difficult for reasons that are familiar to us all. A warm, pleasant and emotionally comforting sensation arises when whenever eat sweets.

Treatments for Tremors

By way of helping people find healthy alternatives that taste as good as sweets with sugar, I aired a radio show[47] with guest Bruce Fife, ND, author of amazing books on cooking with coconut oil, coconut flour and – get this – coconut sugar. Listen to my radio show with Dr. Fife. It will inspire you to change your bad eating habits. You and I well know that it is more important to sedate the tremors (which are a constant nuisance for most people) than it is to enjoy a few minutes of pleasure from eating sweets that are loaded of the sugar toxin.

Certain foods have a beneficial impact on calming tremors. The two leaders in research in discovering recipes and foods that reverse Parkinson's symptoms are Aunt Bean and Glen Pettibone. Together they shared their recent discoveries and recipes on a Parkinsons Recovery Sunday Connections program. Both were diagnosed with Parkinson's disease. Both independently decided to investigate how they could reverse their own symptoms through nutrition. I consider these two remarkable individuals to be the top researchers in the field. Their credentials are impeccable.

---

[47] http://www.blogtalkradio.com/parkinsons-recovery/2014/10/22/reversing-parkinsons-with-coconut-oil

© Parkinsons Recovery

Treatments for Tremors

Actually they were not only the researchers. They become the research subjects of their own discoveries. Be sure to listen to the recording of the Parkinsons Recovery Sunday Connections program[48] for an update on their latest discoveries.

Aunt Bean's Fava Bean Tincture

Aunt Bean has a small farm in Tennessee. She is now famous for her discovery of a fava bean tincture that offers relief from her own tremors. No, you cannot purchase the tincture from her. She makes enough of the tincture to treat only her own Parkinson's symptoms and those of her friends.

The recipe for Aunt Bean's Fava Bean tincture is not a trade secret! She has released a handbook titled "Natural L-Dopa Supplementation You Can Make in Your Own Kitchen." Aunt Bean includes a detailed, step by step explanation on how you can make the fava bean tincture yourself in your own home. To claim the free Fava Bean Recipe handbook, visit the fava beans website maintained by Parkinsons Recovery.[49] Click on the image on the right

---

[48] http://iTeleseminar.com/68356731
[49] http://www.favabeans.parkinsonsrecovery.com

86

© Parkinsons Recovery

column of the main page to download the PDF of her free handbook. You will encounter other recipes that help to calm tremors including L-Dopa Fava Sprout Balls and Fava Pod Juice. Don't those foods sound fun to prepare in your kitchen? They certainly do not require a doctor's prescription.

Glen Pettibone's Solanaceous Vegetables

Glen Pettibone was not having success treating his symptoms with the standard dosage of medications prescribed after his initial diagnosis. He began taking higher and higher doses of his Parkinson's medications at the recommendation of his doctor, but higher doses also did not help. His doctors recommended Deep Brain Stimulation surgery (DBS) as a next step.

Instead of getting DBS, Glen decided to conduct his own research. He intuited that there had to be solutions other than medications that had side effects. One of his fascinating discoveries was that nicotine has been found in some research studies to facilitate the production of dopamine in the body. Of course, smoking is not a viable option given the health risks. Instead of smoking, he drew on his background in science, agriculture, engineering and gardening to identify food that contained high levels of dopamine. The category of food that meets this requirement is known as solanaceous vegetables.

Eggplant found its way to the top of his list of solanaceous vegetables that are high in nicotine content. Glen experimented with a number of ways to eat eggplant. Eating it did not help a great deal. Instead of cooking it, he discovered that he could freeze Chinese eggplant (which is high in nicotine), grate it and then add the grated eggplant to yogurt. This alone apparently helped provide relief from his symptoms.

Glen pursued a comprehensive diet in addition to eating solanaceous vegetables like uncooked eggplant with yogurt. Glen also changed his diet by adding foods that were high in antioxidants like cherries and blueberries.

The result? He succeeded in weaning off all of his medications (though an unfortunate automobile accident created a little burp in his recovery program). Listen to my radio show interview with Glen where you will get the full details on his fascinating discoveries.[50] He has also published a Kindle book that summarizes his discoveries: *Powerful Food and a Walk in the Sun: Parkinson's Relief was in the Supermarket.*[51]

Reversal of symptoms happens when you are in the driver's seat. Make it so today. Why not sprout a bowl of fava beans or prepare some of Glen's Chinese eggplant with yogurt? Follow their recipes and see what happens with your tremors. These food preparations helped them. Maybe they are solutions for you too, eh?

Hydration

Toxins contribute to tremors. You may have pursued a number of detox therapies, but found yourself disappointed they did not calm your tremor. Why not?

The answer is obvious but seldom acknowledged. Your cells are dehydrated. How can your body discharge toxins from cells if there is insufficient fluid? Success is only

---

[50] http://www.blogtalkradio.com/parkinsons-recovery/2014/03/11/parkinsons-relief-was-in-the-supermarket-for-glen-pettibone

[51] http://www.amazon.com/gp/product/B00MEBATMW/ref=as_li_tl?ie=UTF8&camp=1789&creative=9325&creativeASIN=B00MEBATMW&linkCode=as2&tag=zerpoihea-20&linkId=NZ6AWCOIG7KYGV6I

possible when cells are well hydrated. It takes fluid to eliminate the toxins. They do not ooze out on their own.

Jaroslav Boublik PhD is an international expert on hydration and one of the two developers of the Aqua hydration formulas[52]. Dr. Boublik answered a series of important questions about hydration on my radio show[53]. Listen to the recording of this show and marvel at his answers.

Set the intention to insure that your cells are adequately hydrated. You will be amazed at how this little step can help you feel so much better in the long run.

Relax with Aroma Therapy

There are several essential oils with aroma therapeutic properties that suppress tremors. Essential oils are an extremely useful and too often neglected therapy. They reduce persistent levels of stress and anxiety that are the underlying triggers for tremors. As you are well aware, when stress levels skyrocket, tremors worsen. Essential

---

[52] http://www.aquas4life.com

[53] http://www.blogtalkradio.com/parkinsons-recovery/2009/06/04/pioneers-of-recovery

oils calm stress levels. They comfort the body, mind and soul.

Many people are overwhelmed with the essential oil choices that are available. You obviously do not want to try all of them, nor would that be advisable. Which ones should you consider trying?

One way to decide is to solicit informed suggestions from a qualified aroma therapist. Jean Oswald[54], registered nurse and aroma therapist, has years of experience with recommending essential oils that provide relief from symptoms of one form or another. Her consultations (which she offers by telephone) are inexpensive and, I might, add well worth the expense. She has experience working with persons who currently experience Parkinson's symptoms.

Jean is a distributor of Young Living Essential Oils[55] which manufactures high grade and superior quality essential oils. Oils available from other sources may have questionable quality. I have used the Young Living

---

[54] http://www.compassionateconsulting.com

[55] https://www.youngliving.com/en_US/discover/guide/about

Treatments for Tremors

Essential Oils myself. They have often proved beneficial and useful.

Neuro-Auricular Technique (NAT)

Of course, you can dive in and purchase essential oils yourself directly from Young Living Essential oils without getting a consultation from Jean Oswald or another aroma therapist. If you are one of those people who prefers to "dive in" and test the waters so to speak, consider making an appointment with an essential oil massage therapist who is experienced in doing Neuro-Auricular Technique or (NAT). Gary Young, the original founder of the Young Essential Oils, has developed this particular treatment protocol for persons who currently experience neurological symptoms.

The NAT treatment rewires and reconnects the synapses in the brain and upper spine. How cool is that? Essential oil blends are applied along the base of the skull, on the back of neck and down the spine. The NAT treatment protocol uses Frankincense and the Young Living blends RutaVaLa, Valor and Stress Away. The application and treatment of this unique combination of essential oils helps to heal nerve centers and neural pathways that have been torn or

© Parkinsons Recovery

otherwise damaged. Neurological disorders including tremors that originate from these centers can potentially benefit from NAT.

I have personally experienced the NAT treatment and can report it works wonders. Contact an essential oil technician or aroma therapist who has experience and training in offering a NAT therapeutic treatment to their patients. Discuss with them the possibility of getting a NAT treatment for yourself.

I first learned about this therapy from watching a YouTube video of a wife who applied the oils on her husband's back following the NAT protocol. Her husband had been diagnosed with Parkinson's. The video is no longer available on YouTube, but I had the opportunity to discuss this couple's experience at length during a cruise to Alaska that I sponsored through Parkinsons Recovery. I can say with confidence that this therapy provided sustained relief to this man who had advanced symptoms. Once learned, it is a therapy that can be applied frequently by a spouse or friend with continued positive results.

Treatments for Tremors

Putting aside the more comprehensive NAT therapy, specific essential oils can also be beneficial including Frankincense, Basil and the Young Living blends of Stress Away and RutaVaLa. These are previewed next.

Frankincense

Have you ever smelled Frankincense? It has a sweet, comforting aroma that elevates clarity and provides the companion benefit of reducing stress and anxiety. Many people rub it on the bottom of their feet to disperse nervous energy which inevitably causes tremors to escalate.

Basil

Basil is well known for its anti-spasmodic action. It is also considered a traditional treatment for stress.

Stress Away

This Young Living blend was developed to help a person combat the day to day stresses that are unavoidable for everyone. It resets the body's natural ability to relax and releases nervous tensions that enflame tremors. The blend includes vanilla, cedarwood, copaiba, lavender in addition to other complementary oils.

© Parkinsons Recovery

Treatments for Tremors

RutaVaLa

RutaVaLa, another Young Living blend of several essential oils, oxygenates cells in the brain. It also helps to correct misinformation at the cellular level. Apply it to the back of the neck, along the spine, on the soles of the feet or under the nose to calm unpleasant feelings that sustain persistent life stresses. RutaVaLa contains valerian which is one of the herbs used by herbalist Andrew Bentley to treat tremors.

Take Medicine by Ear

The power of sound to sedate tremors is huge! Research is not necessary to convince you this is true, right? Haven't you noticed that your tremors are calmed when you listen to music that resonates with you?

We all know what it means to take "Medicine by Mouth" in the form of pills. Medicine in the form of sound frequencies can also be delivered to our bodies through our ears. Dr. Suzanne Jonas calls this unique and powerful therapy "Medicine by Ear." The guiding principle that inspired Dr. Jonas' formulations is that certain frequencies

© Parkinsons Recovery

Treatments for Tremors

help to heal specific imbalances. The imbalance that is our primary concern is tremors.

Four options for getting medicine by ear that have helped some people reverse tremors are listed next: Dr. Jonas's Parkinson's CDs, Hemi-Sync®, Holosync® and chanting.

Parkinsons CD's

Dr. Suzanne Jonas has mastered two **Parkinson's Disease** CDs that contain highly specific frequencies that were formulated to assist in decreasing the symptoms of Parkinson's Disease including tremors.

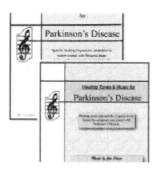

Unique programming embeds pulsed frequencies in nature sounds. She also added binaural beats to assist with faster delivery and enhanced relaxation. The companion CD for Parkinson's contains the same highly specific frequencies

© Parkinsons Recovery

that are embedded in healing music composed by Jim Oliver.

The Parkinson's disease CD was found to be effective in reducing Parkinson's symptoms in a study conducted by researchers at Rush University Medical Center in Chicago. The Rush study found that 23 subjects with a diagnosis of Parkinson's disease experienced a reduction in motor function symptoms after listening for 30 minutes to the Parkinson's CDs every day for 30 days. I ask Dr. Jonas why the research would have revealed such a remarkable result. Her response was fascinating.

She explained that one of the frequencies in her Parkinson's CD is the Schumann resonance which, as you may know, is a unique set of low frequencies that are emitted from the earth's electromagnetic field. When a person is exposed to the Schumann frequencies they become more balanced and centered.

The value of getting exposure to the Schumann frequencies was discovered during the early years of space exploration. When astronauts returned to earth they

© Parkinsons Recovery

found it to be extremely difficult to walk once they landed. NASA solved this problem by playing Schumann resonances in the space capsule while astronauts traveled in space. This solved the problem of wobbliness and sidelined potential embarrassment for NASA. When astronauts now return to earth, they no longer appear to have been drinking on the job.

Listening to the Schumann resonances worked for the astronauts. And, research suggests it is also working for people who currently experience symptoms of Parkinson's too! For more information about Dr. Jonas Parkinson's CD visit the website listed in the footnote here.[56]

Hemi-Sync®

"Hemi-Sync® is a scientifically based and clinically proven "audio-guidance" technology that uses sound to influence brain wave activity. This patented, highly sophisticated technology is backed by over 50 years of development and has been researched extensively at the Monroe Institute[57] in Virginia USA.

---

[56] http://www.frequencymedicine.us

[57] https://www.monroeinstitute.org

Treatments for Tremors

Hemi-Sync® is an audio-guidance process that works through the generation of complex, multilayered audio signals that act in combination to create unique brain wave forms characteristic of specific states of consciousness. The result is a focused, whole-brain state known as hemispheric synchronization or "Hemi-Sync®." The left and right hemispheres of the brain work together in a state of coherence when listening to Hemi-Sync® frequencies.

As an analogy, lasers produce focused, coherent light. Hemi-Sync®[58] produces a focused, coherent mind and facilitates the optimal conditions for stabilizing and centering the body.

Holosync®

Bill Harris has built on the research at the Monroe Institute by developing his own version of sound therapy. He calls his system Holosync®.[59] A demonstration of his sound therapy is available on his website. Bill writes on his website that:

---

[58] https://www.monroeinstitute.org

[59] https://www.centerpointe.com/v2/

Treatments for Tremors

"After nearly three decades of our own research and experimentation, we've created a powerful audio technology called Holosync®, which we place inaudibly beneath peaceful music and environmental sounds. Some call it "instant meditation," but it's much more than that.

Experiencing these deep meditative states each day provides a super-enriched environment for your nervous system, causing enormous (and very beneficial) changes in the brain. What we're actually doing is (gradually) giving the nervous system more input (of a very precise nature) than it can handle... that is, the way it's currently structured... in much the same way exercise gives your body more than it can handle physically, pushing it to grow stronger."

To benefit from this sound therapy you have to use headphones. Frequencies emitted through the right headphone are offset or slightly different from the frequencies emitted from the left headphone. The brain is challenged with forging new neural connections to make sense out of the difference in frequencies that are

© Parkinsons Recovery

received in the right and left sides of the brain. The Centerpointe company developed a series of CDs that increase the spread between the sounds to the right and left ears, respectively.

Several years ago I purchased four sets of the Centerpointe CDs and listened to them in the evening while going to sleep. You do not have to be awake to get the benefit. The benefit to me was a gradual reduction in the extent to which I became over excited, over stimulated and stressed over minor, day to day irritations and unpleasant circumstances. Instead of getting worked up over a driver who gives me the finger because I am driving too slowly, I now allow the insult to wash through me without creating undue stress. In other words, the little stuff no longer pushed me over the edge.

While I did benefit from using this technology – though the benefits took months to be realized – I was put off by the company's aggressive marketing of the product. Once you buy the first CD, they send a ton of mail advertisements to sell you on purchasing the next level of Holosync®. I did purchase four sets but I eventually disengaged from the company. It still is a resource worth considering. I recommend at a minimum that you listen to the sample audio on his website to experience the effects of this form of sound therapy. That will give you an experiential sense of the therapy.

Chant

The Chinese believe that certain sounds create vibrations in the tissues of the body that heal illness from the inside-out. When you realize tremors are fueled by too much energy rushing through the meridians of the body, chanting certain sounds offers a convenient opportunity to dissipate the excess.

Check out Dr. Sha's website[60] as well as his book, *Soul, Mind Body Medicine*[61] to get a handle on this fascinating therapy that only you can do for yourself. If you have always liked to sing, this is surely an option you need to put high on the list of therapeutic priorities to calm your tremor.

---

[60] http://www.drsha.com

[61] http://www.amazon.com/gp/product/1577315286/ref=as_li_tf_tl?ie=UTF8&tag=zerpoihea-20&linkCode=as2&camp=217145&creative=399377&creativeASIN=1577315286

Treatments for Tremors

Vibrate Your Body

Most people use a variety of clever strategies to hide tremors. They:

- Sit on both hands.
- Clasp both hands together tightly.
- Put a hand with the tremor in a pocket.
- Hold a hand with the tremor behind their back.

One approach that has succeeded for some people is to do the reverse: Exaggerate the tremor rather than hide it. Recall that professional Dancer Pamela Quinn, diagnosed with Parkinson's disease, discovered that when her left hand was tremoring, she could calm it down by shaking it vigorously. Why not try shaking a hand or a foot when your tremor becomes troublesome?

Three therapeutic options other than simply shaking an appendage or your entire body can also be explored. The first option involves purchasing vibration technology that does the shaking for you. This method is known as vibration therapy. When sound is added to vibration the therapy is called VibroAcoustic therapy which incorporates the benefits of vibration therapy (Vibro) with sound therapy (Acoustic). Vibration therapy or VibroAcoustic therapy is particularly useful for people who have very low energy and little motivation to help themselves get well.

The other significant benefit of either therapy is that everyone in the family can benefit. The combination of vibration with sound (or vibration alone) pumps up the energy level for everyone who uses it.

Intentional shaking is a second therapy that I recommend you consider. In contrast to VibroAcoustic therapy, it does require that you have enough energy to induce shaking in your own body. Both approaches work directly with tension that is trapped in the physical body. Both release that tension, but in different ways.

The third therapy I highly recommend is to laugh out loud. Anyone can laugh anytime of the day or night. Each of these three therapies is discussed next.

VibroAcoustic Therapy

VibroAcoustic Therapy is delivered with equipment that shakes or vibrates the body while you listen to binaural frequencies through headphones. The proposition that vibration helps reduce symptoms of Parkinson's disease

Treatments for Tremors

was originally hypothesized by Dr. Charcot in the late 1800's. He observed that his patients who came to him after riding in a train or carriage had fewer symptoms than patients who arrived by other means. He theorized that the difference could be explained by the fact that vibration of the people riding in the carriages and trains helped reduce the symptoms.

Dr. Charot actually invented a vibrating chair that was driven by a steam engine. He died in 1893 before the results of his experiment could be evaluated formally and published.[62] The proposition that vibration helps sedate tremors has been re-discovered over the past decade.

The idea of adding sound to vibration is an even more recent discovery. Information about a VibroAcoustic therapy that has proven useful for people with Parkinson's symptoms can be found on the Parkinsons Recovery VibroAcoustic website.[63] The CDs that are included in the

[62] *Dr. Charcot was the medical doctor who is credited with naming the neurological condition that is known today as Parkinson's disease.*

[63] http://www.vibroacoustic.parkinsonsrecovery.com

Treatments for Tremors

VibroAcoustic system described in this website were mastered by Dr. Suzanne Jonas and are the same CDs discussed here under the "Take Medicine by Ear" chapter of this book. The CDs were mastered to assist with all Parkinson's symptoms, not tremors exclusively. As noted previously, Dr. Jonas's CDs contain highly specific frequencies that assist in decreasing the symptoms of Parkinson's disease. The sounds on her Parkinson's CDs embed binaural technology to facilitate the establishment of new neural pathways. Companion benefits are greater relaxation and less stress.

Intentional Shaking

TRE® stands for Tension & Trauma Release Exercise.[64] It is an innovative therapy that involves the deliberate intention to shake your body. I know. I know. You are already shaking enough! The interest here is in sedating the tremors, not empowering them. Why in the world would I recommend that you induce more tremoring voluntarily? You have enough involuntary tremoring already. Right?

---

[64] http://traumaprevention.com

Treatments for Tremors

The reason shaking helps calm tremors is counterintuitive. Tension & Trauma Release Exercises help release patterns of stress, tension and trauma that have embedded in the muscles, tissues and fascia. TRE® activates a natural reflex mechanism of shaking that discharges tension and calms the neurological system. Animals shake to release stress. Humans can do the same. The method provides a pressure relief value for tension and stress.

Laughing

When you laugh out loud, your body shakes. And, as you now know, when your body shakes it manufactures dopamine. It is the natural way to infuse your tissues with a rush of dopamine. How delicious is that?

Laughter Yoga Instructor Gita Fendelman[65] reports that Laughter Yoga helps her get remarkable relief from her own Parkinson's symptoms. This may seem strange, but you learn how to start laughing even though no joke has been told. Laughter instructors like Gita Fendelman teach their students how to induce laughter and as a result, encourage the body to make more dopamine. It is probably the most effective, cheapest and readily available

---

[65] http://www.youtube.com/watch?v=ODv4fgGz4aE

© Parkinsons Recovery

therapy you can practice. All you need is your body which happens to be a resource that is always close at hand! You do not have to go looking for it when you need it.

Activate the Power of Your Mind

Everyone knows that we use a tiny fraction of our minds. Why not access the excess capacity to calm your tremors? This is what Gord Summer does. Gord did not learn how to use the power of his mind to calm his tremors from taking a course on "How to Calm Your Tremor." No, he figured it out all by himself. Being a black belt martial artist helped.

His techniques required that the tremor is dominant on one side of the body and not the other as is the case with many persons who have been diagnosed with Parkinson's disease. The idea in a nutshell is to send the unobstructed energy running through his "good hand" – the one without a tremor - to the hand with the tremor. He channels the strength of his strong side over to the weak side using intention, focus and breath.

Gord was a guest on the Parkinsons Recovery Radio[66] and demonstrates in this video[67] taken at the first Parkinsons

Treatments for Tremors

Recovery Summit in Vancouver how he uses the power of his mind and his martial arts skills to calm his own tremor. Gord's methods are powerful, simple and natural. They also require no special martial arts training or background. All that is needed is a little practice activating the power of the mind to transfer good energy on one side of the body to the other side that is symptomatic.

Transform Beliefs that Inflame Tremors

Some people on the road to recovery succeed temporarily with calming their tremors within a few weeks or months, but eventually revert back to having problems. Recovery for other people is much slower. Still other people plateau and cannot seem to wiggle their way out of tremors that continue to be problematic.

People who have repeated success with sedating their tremors have a special ability to be positive and upbeat. They are convinced that anything is possible. Of course a

---

[66] http://www.blogtalkradio.com/parkinsons-recovery/2010/12/29/now-more-active-than-ever

[67] http://www.blog.parkinsonsrecovery.com/category/power-of-the-mind/

Treatments for Tremors

tremor can be calmed. If a wild animal can be tamed, certainly a tremor can too.

An underlying factor that aggravates tremors is the tendency to recycle negative thought patterns day in and day out. Negative thoughts fertilize the tremors. Too often, negative and destructive thoughts are not even conscious! They whisper at us so quietly we cannot quite make them out. Of course, our subconscious always hears and remembers them.

I wrote *Five Steps to Recovery*[68] to help transform the negative thought patterns that are difficult for all of us to shake off. When I saw how much these five steps helped transform my own thinking I knew they would have a profound impact on others. Once the negative thinking is transformed, great strides in recovery are possible. Transform a tendency to be pessimistic into a preference for optimism and the door is wide open for tremors to be sedated.

---

[68] http://www.fivestepstorecovery.com

© Parkinsons Recovery

Treatments for Tremors

How Long Will It Take for Me to Get Results?

My answer to this question is inspired by interviews with Naturopath John Coleman from Australia. John reversed his Parkinson's symptoms using a variety of therapies. When I asked John what he would recommend to help sedate a tremor, he said that the tremors were the last symptom a person with Parkinson's should be concerned about.

Why I asked? After all, tremors are one of the most visible and embarrassing of all neurological symptoms. John explained that his own tremor was the last symptom to reverse. In fact, John said that his tremors actually got a great deal worse before they got better.

> "My major advice is don't worry about your tremor. Get well. Then the tremor will disappear."

There is a reason why tremors might be the last symptom to be healed. The body prioritizes the energy it allocates to healing various imbalances. The most life threatening and serious problems are addressed first. Tremors are not a life threatening problem, so the body makes the rational choice to attend to other problems first. If tremors are not

© Parkinsons Recovery

Treatments for Tremors

your only symptom, it is most likely that other symptoms and imbalances will be resolved before your tremors are sedated. In short, it may take time and a large dose of patience before you can celebrate having a steady hand and a calm body to accompany a pursuit of your heart felt dreams.

A solution awaits you. Your task is to find the options that will yield results. You obviously cannot take action on all of the suggestions you have now encountered in *Treatments for Tremors.* Which ones call out to you?

May you explore at least one of the possibilities you have encountered while reading this book. If you experiment with several options, you will likely get the best results. Most importantly, may you celebrate the outcome of taking positive action as you sit proudly in the driver's seat of your journey down the road to recovery.

Resources

Free Parkinsons Recovery Newsletter
Do you want to receive notices about the Parkinsons

Recovery radio programs, access to the Sunday

Connections programs and other research updates? Be

sure to sign up for the free Parkinsons Recovery

newsletter.

http://robert_12.subscribemenow.com

Parkinsons Recovery YouTube Videos
I post brief videos that provide information about my

discoveries after more than a decade of research on

Parkinson's disease.

https://www.youtube.com/user/robert7722

Consultations

- Are you confused and perplexed by the many
  options that are available to sedate your tremor?
- Have you tried one or several of the options
  presented in this book and were disappointed in
  the outcome?

Treatments for Tremors

- Are you confused about which way to turn and what options to consider next?

http://www.parkinsonsrecovery.us

Jump Start to Recovery

The focus I have placed in *Treatments for Tremors* has been on sedating them. Are you interested in a longer term solution, one that heals the tremors from the inside-out?

http://www.jumpstart.parkinsonsrecovery.com

Parkinsons Recovery Membership

Would day in and day out support for your recovery be useful? By way of habit, do you use your computer every day? Check out a Parkinsons Recovery Membership.

http://www.parkinsonsrecovery.org

50624658R00066

Made in the USA
San Bernardino, CA
28 June 2017